SHIPWRECKS AROUND ANGLESEY
by
Tom Bennett

Contents — Page

Shipwrecks before 1800, Early wrecks and wreckers	3
Shipwrecks from 1800 to 1850	7
Early steamship wrecks	9
Shipwrecks from 1850 to 1900	14
Shipwrecks since 1900	21
Lifeboats and Lifeboatmen	26
Wreck List	29
Book List	32

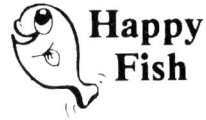
Happy Fish

Reverend Owen Williams, Coxswain of the Cemlyn Lifeboat. His parents devoted their lives to the establishment of six Lifeboat stations around the Anglesey coast. Coxswain Williams was involved with the rescue of passengers from the wreck of the OLINDA in 1854.
(National Lib rary of Wales)

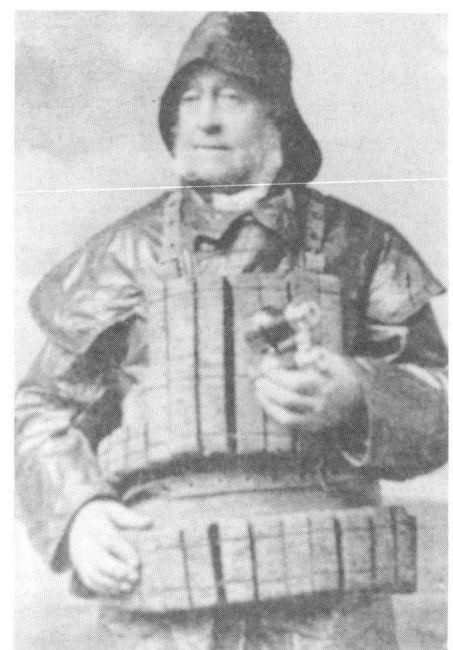

Cover picture shows author's impression of the PRIMROSE HILL being wrecked in 1900.
(See story on page 21).

First Published in 1995 by Happy Fish,
Holmws, Newport, Dyfed, SA42 0UF.

Cover Design by Tom Bennett
Desktop Publishing by Matthews Design
Printed in Wales by D.Brown & Sons Ltd,
Cowbridge and Bridgend, Glamorgan.

Copyright © Tom Bennett 1995

All Rights Reserved. No part of this publication may be reproduced, stored in a retrieval system, or transmitted in any form or by any means, electronic, mechanical, photocopying, recording or otherwise, without the written permission of the author or publisher.

British Library Cataloguing in Publication Data.
A catalogue record of this book is available from the British Library.

Bennett, Tom, 1947–
Shipwrecks around Anglesey.
1. Shipwrecks–Wales–History
1. Title

ISBN - 0 - 9512114 - 6 - 3

Shipwrecks before 1800 - Early Wrecks & Wreckers

Anglesey is the most north westerly extremity of Wales and is the corner of land around which ships have had to sail in order to reach and depart from the port of Liverpool. The importance of Liverpool to the history of shipping around Wales, and especially Anglesey, cannot be overstated. The port of Liverpool influenced pilotage, signalling stations and other harbour developments including lighthouses around the Anglesey coast. It was mostly Liverpool registered ships that were lost around the coast of Anglesey.

Navigating around Anglesey is hazardous. The northern shore is littered with outlying reefs. These can be avoided by choosing a shorter route through the Menai Straits but knowledge of the shoaling waters and picking the correct time of the tide to enter and depart is essential for a safe passage.

Written accounts of the earliest shipwrecks are not available. St Patrick is said to have been shipwrecked on the north Anglesey shore, where his church now stands at Llanbadrig. Amongst the earliest written accounts of shipwrecks were those involving ferries. In 1325 a ferry with passengers from Beaumaris was wrecked and in 1664 a ferry near Caernarfon met with disaster, 80 people losing their lives. Many thought the disaster a judgement from the Almighty. The ferry had been built with timbers stolen from the disused Llanddwyn church.

Before the two Victorian bridges were built, Telford's Suspension Bridge in 1826, and Brittania Bridge in 1856, all goods and people had to cross to Anglesey by sea transport. The Moel y Don Ferry is known to have been established in the thirteenth century when stone was quarried on the island and taken across the Straits to build the walls of Caernarfon Castle. In October 1710, in rough weather, this ferry sank when carrying 10 horses and 15 men, fortunately all were saved. Thirteen years later a similar catastrophe occurred to the same ferry. This time 30 people died and only two survived, one being a boy who grabbed hold of the tail of a horse that took him to the shore.

The outlying rocks off Holyhead are known as the Skerries, these have been responsible for numerous shipwrecks. Historically, one of the most important was the Royal Yacht MARY which hit the Skerries in a fog in 1675. This 52 foot sloop was the first Royal Yacht, a gift from Amsterdam to Charles II, 35 people out of 74 on board lost their lives when the MARY was wrecked near where the present lighthouse is situated. The wreck site was one of the first to be given designation under the Protection of Wrecks Act. Artifacts from this site including bronze cannon, silver forks, coins, lockets and a pewter chamber pot can be seen at the Liverpool Maritime Museum.

Holyhead has been associated with packet boats to Ireland since the first contracts were made during Charles II's reign. In 1670 the first recorded packet boat from Holyhead was lost together with 120 passengers. In September 1710 the Holyhead packet boat ANN was lost in the Irish Sea and within a month a similar tragedy happened to the PEMBROKE, which disappeared without trace. In 1726 a Bangor ferry was lost in the Straits and another Abermenai passenger boat returning from a fair at Caernarfon in 1785 capsized with the loss of 56 people. There was only one survivor a man named Hugh Williams. Thirty five years later history was to repeat itself, another ferry capsized in the Straits drowning 23, similarly there was one survivor, remarkably his name again was Hugh Williams.

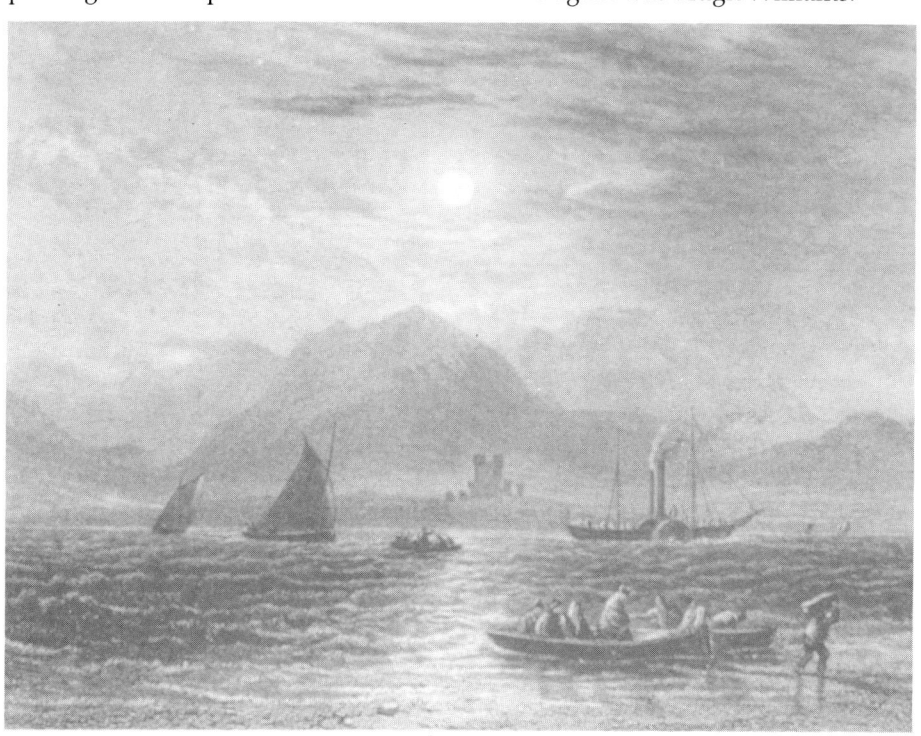

Entrance to the Menai Straits around 1832, this etching shows the Beaumaris ferry and an early paddle steamer. (Tom Bennett Collection)

Liverpool opened its first large dock in 1715 and soon developed to be a leading port in the British Isles. The Liverpool Corporation sought improvements around the coast, lighthouses and coal burning beacons were constructed to identify the hazards. The Skerries had a beacon built upon it by private enterprise in 1716.

As in all remote regions of the British Isles, stories of wreckers abound. Eighteenth century records show that those caught and convicted on Anglesey for "robbing" wrecks were hanged for their crimes.

Lewis Morris, Customs Officer at Holyhead, wrote to the Admiralty in 1741 that *'false charts serve but as false lights laid by villains along ye coast to lead poor sailors to destruction'*. Morris was to carry out detailed chartwork of all the coast of Wales, giving additional recommendations of how each harbour could be improved, and his work formed the basis of the best Welsh charts. Lewis Morris's comments reinforce earlier stories that one wrecker near Newborough used to alter the position of the light at Llanddwyn so that he would have more wrecks to plunder.

A shipwreck that occurred off Carmel Head around 1743 has an interesting conclusion. Two seven year old boys came ashore from the wreck, lashed to a makeshift raft. The identity of the ship, thought to be Spanish, was never established as the boys, speaking a foreign language, were the only survivors. They were fostered in local farms, learnt Welsh and grew up to be eminent members of the community.

The 14 gun frigate ANN was outward bound from Liverpool for the West Indies when a gale hit her in 1760. Unable to weather the storm Captain Houghton decided to run his ship onto the sands near Caernarfon. When his ship struck the sand some abandoned by boat, others swam ashore and some remained. The Captain could not persuade the remainder to leave the ship so, he put on a cork lifejacket, jumped into the sea and went ashore, 18 of the crew drowned and 19 survived. The same gale killed the entire crew of the Liverpool ship PEARL also near Caernarfon. A common grave at Llandwrog was the resting place for 14 that were washed ashore from the two wrecks.

A sloop the "CHARMING JENNY" wrecked as a result of false lights, near Rhosneigr and was robbed by the local people in 1773. Three men, known as *"lladron creigiau Crigyll", the robbers of Crigyll rocks,* were found guilty. On the last day of 1740 the Liverpool brigantine LOVEDAY & BETTY came ashore near Rhosneigr. The Captain secured his vessel and set out overland to get assistance, only to find that when he returned everything that could be carried off had been. Four men were tried at Beaumaris Assizes but to the great consternation of the Captain and others, the men were discharged. Further injustices happened in 1778 when a jury discharged some men accused of robbing another Crigyll wreck named SILCOT. The vessel smashed up on the rocks the majority of the crew and the Captain's wife were drowned. Most of the cargo was stolen by the local people, some were caught in the act. Again justice was not delivered at Beaumaris but, the Captain succeeded in getting some of the men sentenced at Chester Assizes. One of the accused was sent to the gallows and his accomplices transported overseas.

Although criminal and inhuman acts were associated with shipwrecks on the coast of Anglesey in the eighteenth century, the people also showed great acts of humanity and kindness. In 1772 the Druidical Society of Anglesey was founded. One of its objectives was to reward people who saved life at sea. It published in both Welsh and English *'The mode prescribed by the Humane Society for the recovery of persons suspected of being suffocated and drowned'*.

In September 1785 hundreds of barrels and rum puncheons came ashore in Red Wharf Bay. The FAME,

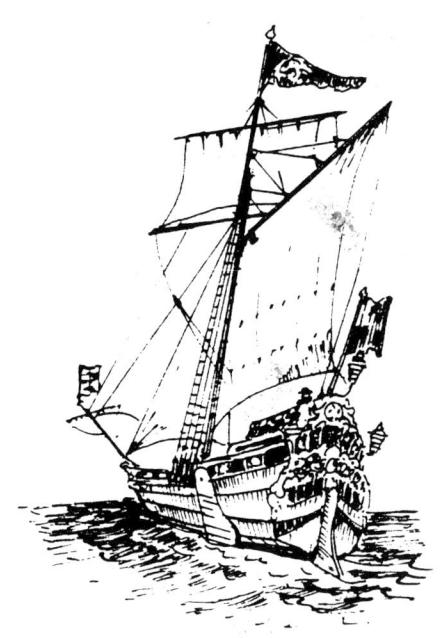

In 1675, before the Skerries Lighthouse guarded the north Anglesey shore, the Royal Yacht MARY ran onto the reefs, half of those on board lost their lives. (Tom Bennett Collection)

from Liverpool to Dublin had been wrecked, 16 men and 3 women had been lost out of 49 on board. According to the Customs officer in Beaumaris the vessel was completely smashed up *"not a plank of any timber together"* and he reported that only 6 puncheons of rum and some deer skins had been recovered. The Times dated 19th October stated *"It is said there was a box of silver on board in bullion, and a considerable sum of specie (coins) together with a very valuable cargo of rum and sugar, all of which, except for a few puncheons of rum, were totally lost"*. Perhaps metal detectors today may be able to locate the riches of the FAME.

Shipwrecks from 1800 to 1850

Unfortunately space does not permit the author to write about all the wrecks as there were in excess of 80 ships lost around Anglesey in the first half of the nineteenth century alone.

The Act of Union of the Parliaments of Great Britain and Ireland in 1800 brought a new importance to the passenger trade entering Holyhead and between 1810 and 1821 the Admiralty Pier, now the car ferry, was constructed.

A red light was constructed at South Stack in 1809 which helped mariners locate the entrance to Holyhead. A north, north easterly gale the same year drove the brig CORNELIA outward from Liverpool to Madeira onto the shore near Holyhead. This ship was lost but some of her cargo was saved. 1819 was a particularly disastrous year for losses around Anglesey. In January the FRIENDSHAFT from Liverpool to Havre was driven onto the shore at Malltraeth, only the chief mate survived. Two weeks later the ship was taken to Beaumaris for repair. The same gale saw the loss of BRANSTE near the Skerries, a ship outward bound from Whitehaven and JANE inward from the West Indies drove ashore in Caernarfon Bay. In November 1819, the vessel WILLING MAID, Liverpool to Bristol was abandoned by her crew off Point Lynas, being in a sinking state. The overloaded Tal y Foel sailing ferry sank in windy conditions in the Menai Straits in 1820, drowning 25 people.

Three years later another passenger boat, the Irish Packet ALERT was sailing past Cemaes Head when the wind dropped . The ship slowly drifted onto the West Mouse (see back cover) where it capsized. Only 7 survived out of 152 on board. The local rector and his wife watched helplessly from the shore, unable to do anything as there was no lifeboat nearby. It so affected the Reverend James Williams and his wife Frances that they devoted their lives to the formation of Anglesey Association for the Preservation of Life from Shipwreck, referred to later in the text as the Anglesey Lifeboat Association or simply as the Association. The Reverend James Williams was justly awarded the very first RNLI Gold medal in Wales after being involved in a rescue of sailors from the vessel ACTIVE that was wrecked in Cemaes Bay in 1835. Using his horse to help him get deeper into the surf, he threw a grappling hook at the wreck and rescued 5 men.

Sometimes ships founder at sea without anyone ashore even knowing about it. Ships leave port and are lost without trace – no survivors to explain what happened. On other occasions, such as in

January 1827, people ashore saw a ship sink but were unable to identify it. The Cambrian newspaper reported that a brig *"with yellow sides of about 140 tons, main boom painted green"* sank with all on board between North and South Stacks, Holyhead. The name of the ship was never ascertained. Present day recreational divers may come up with a named ship's bell that could throw some light on the mystery.

The American barque SARAH came ashore at Trwyn du in 1835. A Beaumaris steamer attempted to tow her off but the barque's bottom had been ripped out and she was not expected to be got off. Petersburgh registered, she was taking 100 tons of salt to New Orleons. A plethora of ships were wrecked near Holyhead in the following two decades. FAME, HARLEQUIN and sloop ACTIVE in 1829. CYGNET in 1830, IPHEGENIA in 1832, GEORGE and MARTHA in 1833 and PLUTARCH a full rigged ship in 1835, sloop JANE and BETTY in 1836, ship PANTHEA New York about 1839, ADELAIDE in Cymyran Bay in 1841.

Captain Williams, Master of the MOUTAINEER knew the Anglesey coast well but he underestimated the strength of an October gale in 1841. The gale drove the full rigged ship onto the North Bank of the Caernarfon Bar. Fortunately the Llanddwyn Lifeboat was on hand to save Captain Williams, his wife, three children and 12 crew. Tragically one crewman

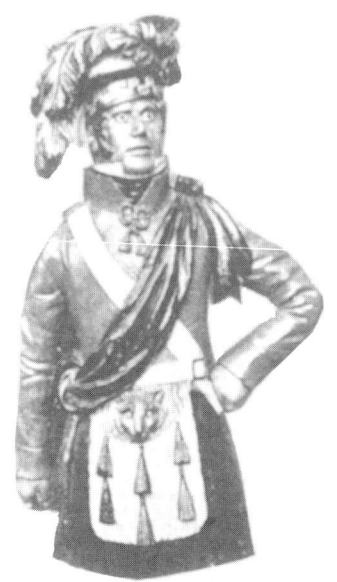

Figurehead of the sailing ship MOUNTAINEER wrecked on the north bank of the Caernarfon Bar in 1841. It stood in the porch at Parkia, home of Sir Llewelyn Turner, who described the figurehead as a "well behaved gentleman".

became entangled in the rigging where he died before he could be rescued. The figurehead was recovered from the wreck and stood for some years in Sir Llewelyn Turner's porch at Parkia, near Caernarfon.

On New Year's Eve 1845 a local lad on the shoreline single handedly managed to saved the ship ALHAMBRA from certain doom. The large ship was seen in trouble heading for the rocks at Rhoscolyn. Realizing the predicament of the ship and understanding the coast the lad swam out to a rock and using his jacket as a flag directed those on board the ship to sail her around the peninsular into the shelter of the bay.

Early Steamship Wrecks

The first steamers were all paddle driven and the first to be lost on the coast of Wales was at Cemaes when the Greenock paddle steamer ROBERT BRUCE was lost in 1820. A regular link between Bangor and Liverpool was commenced in 1822 with an early steamer named ALBION, she was eventually wrecked near Rhyl in 1846.
The most notable of the early steamship losses occurred off Beaumaris in 1831. It was a day trip when everything that could go wrong did go wrong, a rotten and leaky ship, a drunken Captain, no distress signals, inadequate lifeboats and equipment in disrepair. The ROTHSAY CASTLE was making a day trip to Beaumaris which turned out to be a one way trip to hell with over a 100 lives being lost. Departing two hours late caused the leaky ship to have a rougher passage than normal and at midnight they found themselves tossed about on the sands of Dutchman's Bank, the vessel breaking apart beneath them in the shallow water. When the steamer broke apart, all the passengers found themselves in the water, fighting to save their lives. Some climbed onto a piece of wreckage and used one of the lady passenger's petticoats as a distress flag, they were the lucky ones and were rescued, but 107 others were drowned. Lessons were learnt and it prompted compulsory signalling equipment to be carried on all such vessels.

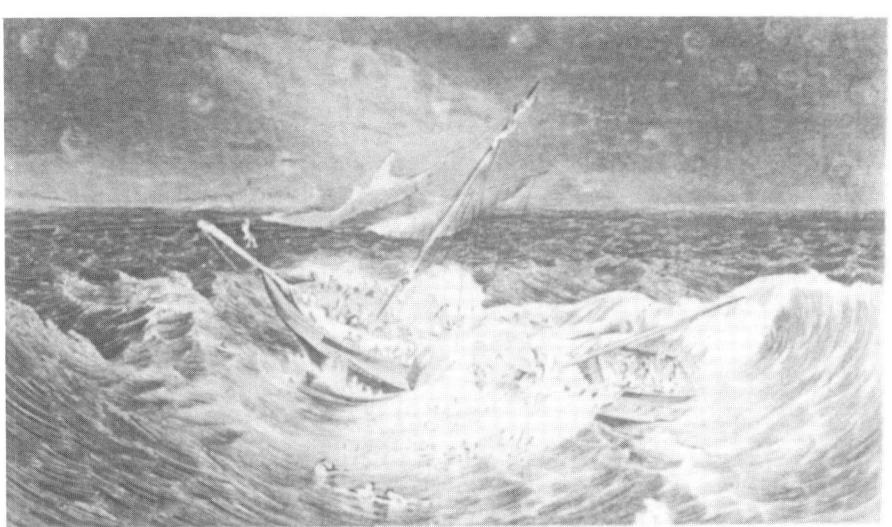

A day trip to Beaumaris in 1831 turned into a nightmare when the paddle steamer ROTHSAY CASTLE broke up on the Dutchman's Bank. Over 100 people were drowned. This incident prompted legislation for ships to carry a means of signalling distress at night. (Tom Bennett collection)

Ships carrying emigrants to America have been lost around the North Wales coast often causing terrible loss of life. The steamship NOTTINGHAM collided with the barque GOVERNOR FENNER in 1841 causing the loss of 122 lives, mostly emigrants on their way to New York.

Some poor decisions by the Captain of a wooden paddle steamer MONK in 1843 were to cause the loss of his ship, his life and the lives of 18 other people. He commenced a voyage from Porthdinllaen to Liverpool with a cargo of butter and 140 pigs. Missing the tide he still attempted to enter the Menai Straits when, in the windy conditions, the steerage would not respond. The small steamer stranded, 3 escaped in the ship's boat and alerted the Llanddwyn Lifeboat which succeeded in saving 2 people as the wreck broke apart. The others were lost including the Captain who was found washed up surrounded by drowned pigs on a beach near Fort Belan.

January 1868 was a busy month for the local Coastguards. They saved the crew of the Boston barque ATLANTIC when the ship came ashore at Aberffraw, unlike the previous month when the capsized EUPHRATES came ashore in the same area, drowning all her crew. Bad weather hit the TOWN OF WEXFORD, steaming from her home port to Liverpool with passengers and a cargo of livestock. Those on land noticed that she was labouring heavily and was under sail when off the Skerries. She anchored in Holyhead Bay but her anchor parted and she came ashore at Trefadog. The Lifeboat crew at Holyhead had anticipated her fate and using a local tug to tow them, helped to save all 43 persons on board. The Cambrian newspaper dated 16th January 1852 states *"..everyone of them was preserved. Little however, was saved of the cargo, as many dead cattle and pigs were seen floating about the bay"*.

Two years later Pilot error caused the loss of the first screw steamer on the notorious reefs off Cemlyn. The North Wales Chronicle condenses the facts. *"The OLINDA, built for the conveyance of passengers and goods to Lisbon and the Brazils..among the best appointed and furnished ships that ever left the British coasts. She was in the charge of an experienced Liverpool pilot, who from some strange fatality, kept close to the Anglesey coast, instead of standing outside the Skerries."*. She struck the reefs inside Harry Furlough's rock. Panic subsided when everyone realized that the ship was grounded but not actually sinking and within an hour all had been taken off into the ship's boats or the Cemlyn Lifeboat. With a severe gash in her hull the OLINDA, less than one year old, was left to the ravages of the sea.

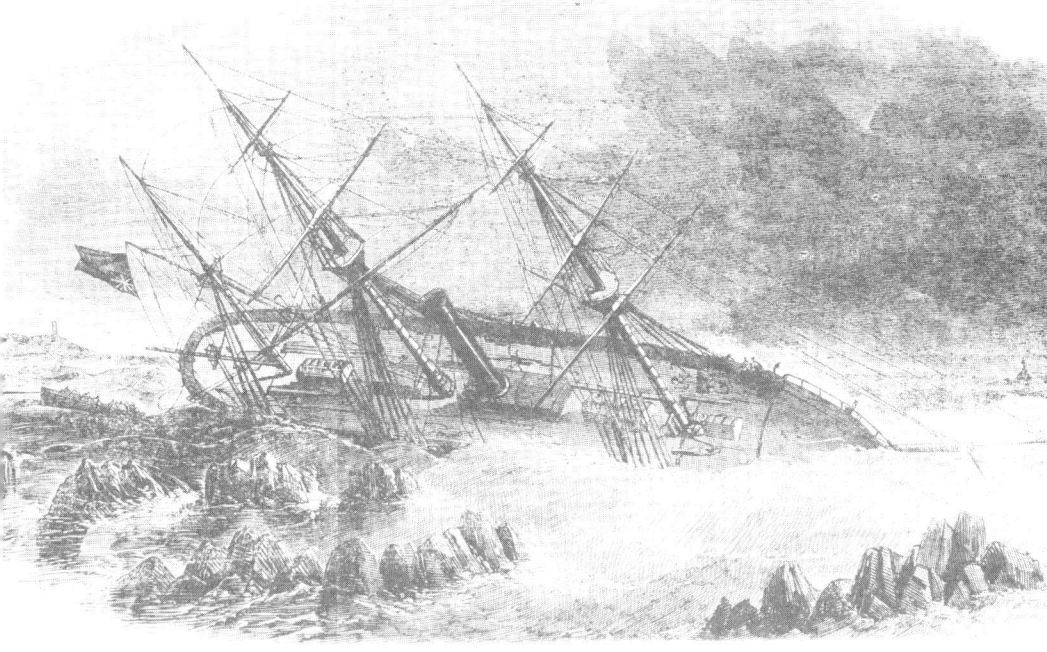

Pilot error caused the barque rigged screw steamer OLINDA to hit Harry Furlough's Reef in 1854. The Cemlyn Lifeboat, seen astern of the wreck, saved the passengers and crew. (Illustrated London News)

Not far away, on Victoria Rock, another steamer was lost later in the same year. Named MINERVA and built in Liverpool for the Cork Steamship Company she had had a chequered history, hitting and sinking two sailing ships in her seven year life and killing at least 7 people. On this occasion her crew and 130 passengers were all rescued. Her Captain may have been to blame. He was also in command of another vessel AJAX that was lost three months later.

The most well known of all Welsh shipwrecks is the ROYAL CHARTER. More than a hundred ships were wrecked around the coast of Wales and about 222 vessels lost around the United Kingdom in just two days of severe storm on the 25th and the 26th October 1859. Over 800 lives were lost, half of them from this one shipwreck the ROYAL CHARTER. Homeward bound from Australia to Liverpool, it was inconceivable that such a luxuriously appointed iron clipper of 2719 tons could be wrecked a few hours journey from her home port. While rounding Anglesey the hurricane turned to east north east. The small 200 horsepower engine and two bladed propeller could do nothing to help keep the large 336 foot iron ship off the rocks near Moelfre. The Moelfre villagers rigged up a bosun's chair to the bowsprit of the wreck. With immense seas showing no mercy, the

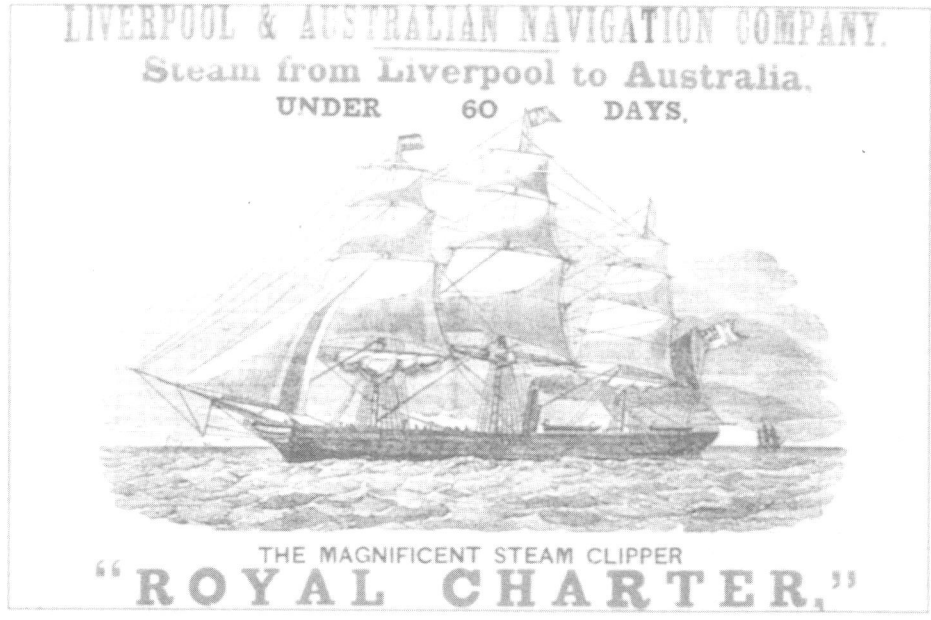

The ROYAL CHARTER from a contemporary poster advertising her voyages to Australia.

women and children refused or were too scared to use this rescue line to the shore. Valuable time was lost and soon the waves, eighteen metres high, smashed the iron hull to pieces. The hull broke apart spilling passengers, crew and cargo into the swirling foam. Passengers with their hard earned sovereigns in their pockets and gold miners returning home with money belts all, unsuccessfully, tried to swim ashore. Most did not make it and no women or children were saved. One man who failed to get ashore alive was found with £320 worth of gold on him that had dragged him to his death.

The writer Charles Dickens visited the wreck site some ten weeks after the event. He watched divers salvaging the wreck of the ROYAL CHARTER, searching for the gold bars and wealth known to have been on board. He wrote " *They are lifting today the gold found yesterday – some £25,000. Of £350,000's worth of gold, £300,000's worth, was at that time recovered.*" Dickens was deeply impressed at the work undertaken by the Vicar of Llanallgo in identifying bodies and replying to no less than 1075 letters of enquiry in ten weeks. Dickens wrote "*The Vicar...worked alone for hours solemnly surrounded by eyes that could not see him, and lips that*

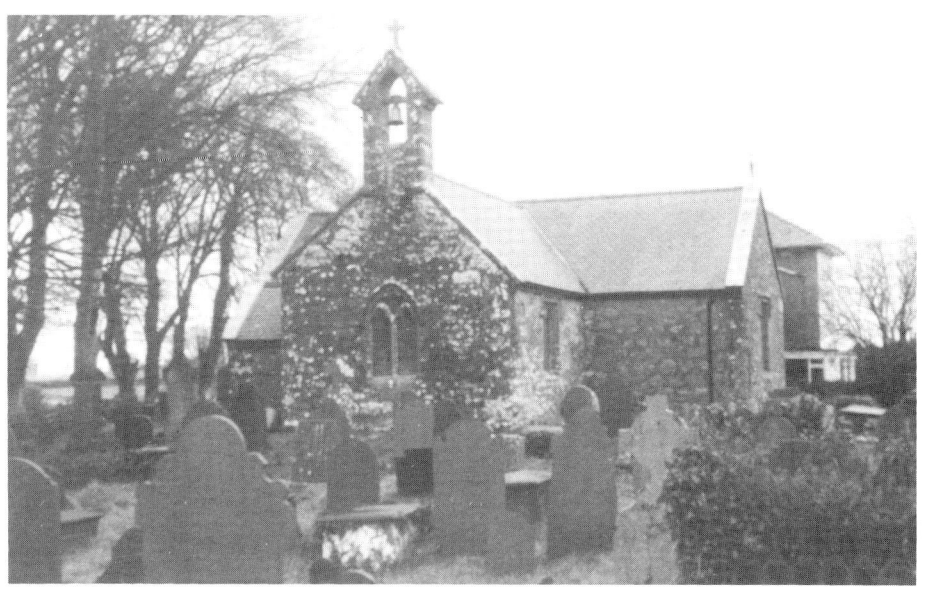

ABOVE - Llanallgo Church, near Moelfre where the victims of the ROYAL CHARTER are buried. Charles Dickens described it as "the little churchyard where so many are so strangely brought together". (Tom Bennett Collection)

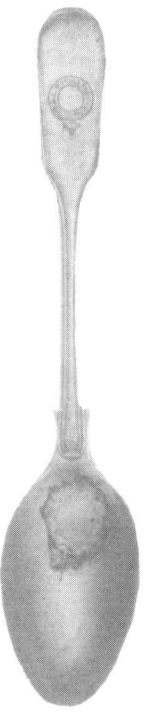

LEFT - A silver teaspoon recovered from the wreck of the ROYAL CHARTER showing the emblem of the Liverpool and Australian Navigation Company. (Tom Bennett Collection)

could not speak to him, patiently examining the tattered clothing, cutting off buttons, hair, marks from linen, anything that might lead to subsequent identification."

Many of the bodies that could not be identified were buried in the churchyard at Llanallgo where a publicly subscribed memorial stone is to be seen.

The sailing barque LA PLATA was starting a voyage to Peru when a white light was spotted ahead one dark night in 1863. The light was thought to be a fixed light on one of the Skerries, but it was actually a steamer on a collision course. When the mistake was realized it was too late. There was a collision, causing both ships to sink but amazingly everyone survived.

Shipwrecks from 1850 to 1900

During the second half of the eighteenth century the greatest numbers of both sailing ships and steamers were lost around the Welsh coast.

In March 1850 an east north east gale wrecked the Liverpool sloop BROTHERS near Penmon. The Captain, his wife and one seaman were drowned. The bodies of the Captain and his wife being found clasped in each others arms on the beach.

In the sands at Malltraeth, a mile north of Llanddwyn Island, are some ribs of a wreck that tell an interesting story. They are the remains of the ATHENA, a greek brig lost there in 1852, whilst carrying a cargo of beans from Alexandria to Liverpool. The Llanddwyn lifeboat was launched but the lifeboatmen failed to row their lifeboat around Llanddwyn Island. Not to be outdone a team of Newborough horses hauled the Lifeboat over the dunes to launch nearer to the wreck. They successfully saved 14 crew. Six days later they saved 9 from the Prussian brig DIE KRONE and the following day saved 13 from the Russian barque JUNO. The RNLI awarded Thanks On Vellum to Hugh Williams, the Coxswain.

The first of the China tea clippers to hit the west coast of Anglesey was the JOHN O'GAUNT. Built at Liverpool in 1835, of 449 tons, she had a reputation for speedy passages to and from China. Unfortunately when she struck the coast near Trearddur in January 1854, all the crew were lost.

The following month the ship BONAVENTURE became dismasted and was driven ashore at Rhosneigr, but the crew fortunately escaped before the wreck broke apart.

The Liverpool ship SOUTHERN CROSS was wrecked at Rhoscolyn Head in March 1855, the 17 crew escaped to a small rock where they had to wait twelve hours before being rescued by the Rhoscolyn Lifeboat.

A force 12 north north west hurricane caused the barque PARMELIA FLOOD to founder off Aberffraw in January 1863. She was carrying a cargo of cotton, oil cake and hides from New Orleans and all her crew drowned except for two. 11 were lost and also one Llanddwyn pilot. One of the survivors was the Captain J A Anderson of New York. He had a miraculous escape holding on to part of the poop when his ship sank and staying with the piece of wreckage for twenty hours in a desperate struggle to stay alive. The wind and currents took him ashore

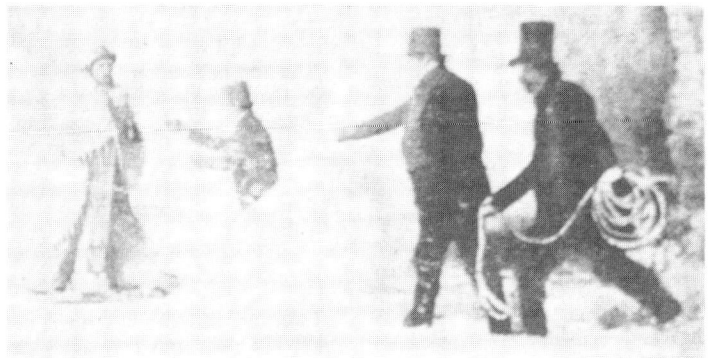

The New York barque PARMELIA FLOOD was wrecked on Caernarfon Bar in 1863. A Llanddwyn Pilot and nearly all the crew were lost. The Captain survived and was washed ashore at Tymawr, where he was photographed with his rescuers on the beach by H J Hughes. (W R Owen)

8 miles south west of Caernarfon where two local men helped him ashore. It is amazing that the Captain survived and it is a coincidence that H J Hughes, the Caernarfon photographer, was there to record the event (see photograph).

The Liverpool sailing ship EARL OF CHESTER, built at Chester in 1845, hit offshore rocks at Rhosneigr in October 1867. The ship was wrecked, the Captain, his wife, the crew and 10 passengers were all lost. The newspapers reported that the Crigyll robbers were out again, preying on the merchandise that washed ashore.

A few months later the barque BAYADERE ran into the rocks near Holyhead Lighthouse. The Holyhead Lifeboat, in a tremendous northerly gale, managed to rescue the crew of 12. They then rowed out to the LYDIA WILLIAMS, 34 were rescued including a woman passenger clutching her young baby.

The Llanelli schooner MERLIN was in collision with a steamer in Holyhead Bay in 1874, and sank within minutes. A dense fog the following year caused the large New York sailing ship NIAGARA to be wrecked on the rocks at Penrhosfeilw. Her cargo was cotton and surprisingly 200 sewing machines.

Also of American interest was the wreck of the steamer ABBOTSFORD, which stranded and sank in 1875 where the Wylfa Power Station now stands. One of the largest steamers to be totally wrecked on the Anglesey coast was the DAKOTA in 1877, 400 feet long and built for speed for the transatlantic run, she was on her way to New York, when an order was given to alter course away from the coast. For some unexplained reason the ship turned the wrong way and headed straight for the coast. The Master, who was near the bow at the time, hurried to the helm to find out what was going on. At fourteen knots it was too late, the liner hit the rocks of the East Mouse and became a wreck, the 218 passengers being ferried ashore by the Bull Bay Lifeboat. The Court of Inquiry suspected an error by the helmsman but those giving evidence all said the wheel was turned correctly although the ship turned the wrong way.

Three years later the sister ship of the DAKOTA, the MONTANA hit Church Bay, opposite Holyhead, in a fog. The Liverpool Daily Post reported *"The passengers were in bed when the vessel struck and only some of them were aroused by the shock"*.... The forward compartment became holed and filled but the sea was smooth and with a falling tide the stranded liner's crew could get passengers into boats without panic. The Lifeboat and a tug was alerted and went across the bay to help, conveying passengers, mail and crew back to Holyhead. The Trinity Steamer tried to tow her off but without success.

Returning from Calcutta the Liverpool iron barque GILBERT THOMPSON was under tow when she hit the West Mouse rock in 1881. Tragically a boy who was lying in his bunk with a broken leg drowned when the ship went down. The remainder of the crew saved themselves and were conveyed to Liverpool by tug boat.

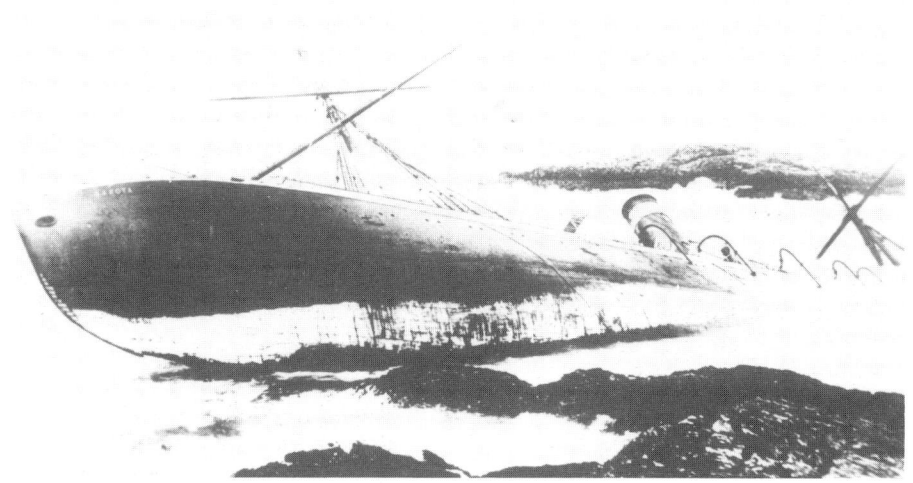

The transatlantic liner DAKOTA was outward bound to New York in 1877 when, for some unknown reason, she turned the wrong way and hit the East Mouse Rock. (Henry Parry Collection, Gwynedd Archives Service XS/1279/S/31)

The efforts of three lifeboat crews combined in a complicated rescue to save the crew of a barque that stranded on Cymyran Beach in March 1883. With a new captain, the NORMAN COURT had a sugar cargo from Java returning to her home port of Greenock when an error in navigation caused her to hit the Crigyll rocks. The Rhosneigr Lifeboat, in huge breakers, tried unsuccessfully to get across Cymyran Bay, after capsizing and breaking equipment she returned. The Holyhead Lifeboat with the aid of a steamer tow got within a mile of the wreck but three attempts to get through the surf failed. Rockets from the shore also failed and so did another attempt by the Rhosneigr Lifeboat. The NORMAN COURT'S crew could be seen in the rigging, desperately clinging on as they were buffeted all night by the waves, 2 died of hypothermia.

The Holyhead crew, after returning, heard that the Rhosneigr Lifeboat had still not been successful in taking people off the wreck. They decided there was still time to perform a rescue. The railway company put on a special train to get the Holyhead crew to Rhosneigr. Using the Rhosneigr Lifeboat the Holyhead crew rowed out in mountainous seas and managed to save 20 from the NORMAN COURT.

A collision between the Holyhead ferry HOLYHEAD and the German barque ALHAMBRA in October 1883, 15 miles off the coast, caused the loss of both vessels and 20 lives including the German Captain and his daughter. The London and North Wales Railway Company lost another ferry the ADMIRAL MOORSOM in similar circumstances when she collided with an American ship and sank off Holyhead in January 1885, losing 5 lives.

The Llanelli barque JAMES KENWAY, built in Canada 13 years earlier, and carrying salt, went ashore three quarters of a mile south of Carmel Head in 1886. The 13 crew abandoned in a boat that then capsized on landing, drowning 2 of them. The Captain, who stayed with the vessel was later rescued by the Holyhead Lifeboat.

The magnificent ship MISSOURI, 5146 tons gross, a steamer with a four masted barque rig, was returning from Massachusetts in 1886. In a driving snowstorm she struck near Porth Dafarch, three miles from her intended course. The crew got off using a breeches buoy but the 426 foot hull refused to be got off with tugs. The hull quickly sank drowning the majority of her cargo of cattle. A hole was blasted through her hull to help salvage the general cargo and various local people were convicted of stealing. The iron parts of her hull still litter the seabed making it one of the most popular shallow dive sites for recreational divers in Anglesey.

Coal Rock near the Skerries was to claim victims in December 1886 with the loss of 11 crew and their 300 ton steamer FAWN. The following year the Glasgow built steamer LORD ATHLUMNEY sank only a few hundred metres away.

Sterling work was done by Coastguard Williams throughout the 1880's in the Holyhead area. His alertness helped in saving 134 crew of the Canadian barque GLEN GRANT when she went on the rocks of Penrhos in 1889.

In 1890, the Liverpool barque HERMINE sailed into Rhoscolyn Bay hit the rocks and quickly went over on her beam ends, the 13 crew clinging on to the sides of the iron ship. Two Lifeboats, a steam tug and a shore boat all raced to the scene but two Rhoscolyn men managed to save all the crew before they arrived.

The crew of the Swedish barque HUDIKSVALL were grateful for the services of a new second Lifeboat to be stationed at Holyhead in 1890. A bold and daring rescue saved all 116 men who had lashed themselves to the upper rails after their ship had crashed into the rocks at Ynys y Fydlyn.

In 1892 the steamer MEATH came ashore at Penrhyn Point. All 32 were saved by the ingenuity and skill of the Holyhead Lifeboat Coxswain Robert Jones, who decided to beach the Lifeboat in order to get the men ashore. Tragically the next day when helping to recover the Lifeboat from Penrhyn beach, Coxswain Jones was injured, injuries from which he later died.

The steamer MERSEY, 342 tons, in the summer of 1894 ran aground close to the Porth Ruffydd Lifeboat Station. The steamer slid off into deeper water, her crew of 13 scrambling ashore by means of a ladder.

A December storm in 1894 caused devastation to shipping in Anglesey. The schooner JOHN WIGNALL sank in Red Wharf Bay and three large vessels were wrecked at Holyhead. Both Holyhead Lifeboats were out all day rescuing shipwrecked crews. At Penrhos the Norwegian barquentine VALHALLA drove ashore, the Lifeboat saving 10 crew. 11 crew were saved later the same day from the Norwegian barque TITANIA in almost the same place. The Liverpool barque KIRKMICHAEL came ashore under bare poles on the Holyhead breakwater. Rescue came from the cliff rescue team who had to crawl along the breakwater, dragging their gear behind them, for fear of being washed away. Fixing a line they rescued 11 men, but 7 crew

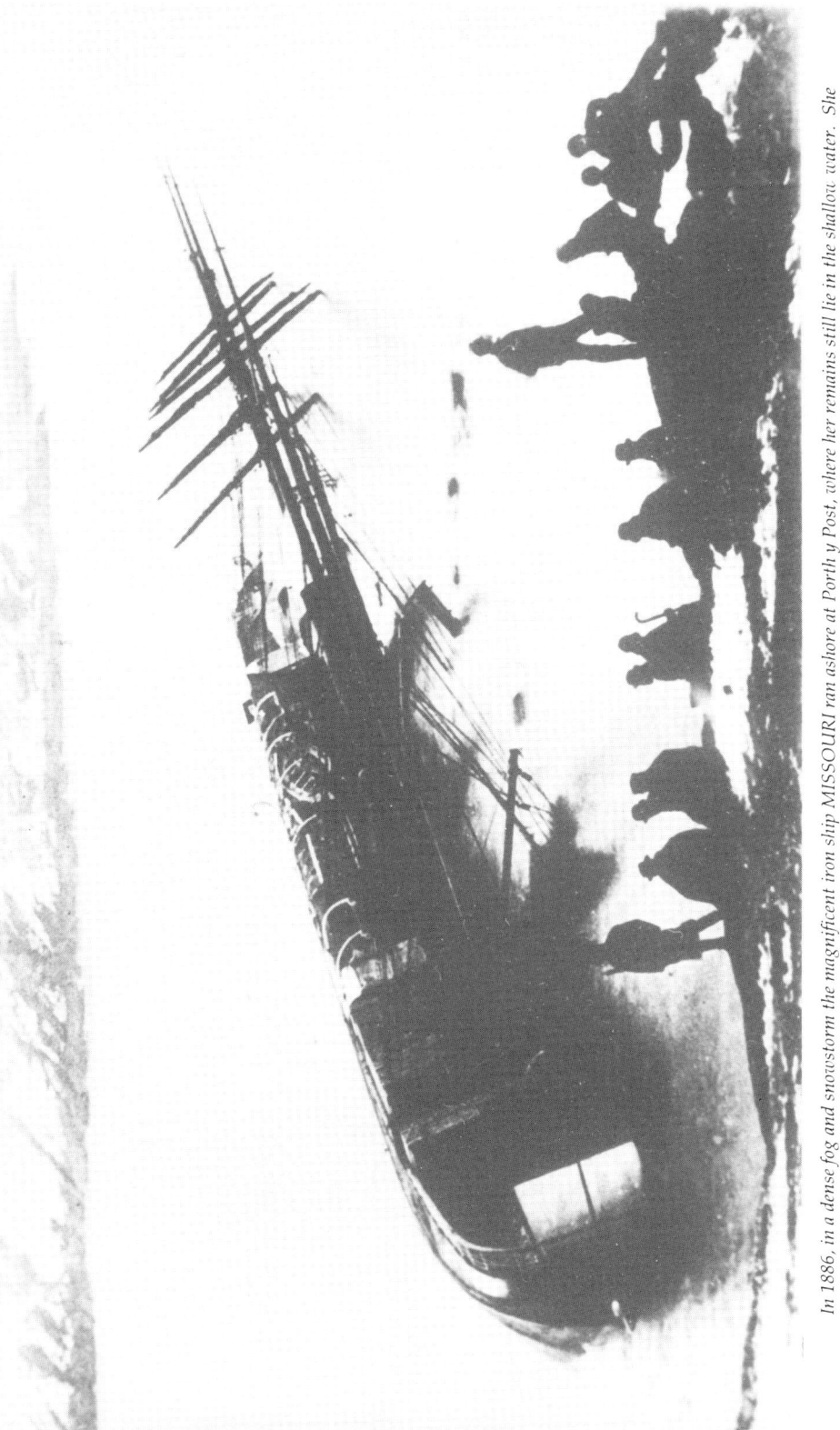

In 1886, in a dense fog and snowstorm the magnificent iron ship MISSOURI ran ashore at Porth y Post, where her remains still lie in the shallow water. She was a 4 masted screw barque of the Warren Line, 5,146 gross tons, 426 feet long with 600 horsepower compound steam engine, built in Glasgow in 1881. (Henry Parry Collection, Gwynedd Archives Service XS/1279/S/32)

were lost. One man stayed aboard, his judgement was correct, because he was found still alive the next morning and was safely landed. The remains of her hull can be seen by divers today on the seabed on the outer side of the breakwater. The following week the barque OSSEO also hit outer breakwater, 1,463 tons and 245 feet long, her entire crew of 26 were drowned.

In 1897 the Dominion Line ANGLOMAN, 4,892 tons, carrying a cargo of 700 American cattle and 1500 sheep, hit the Skerries West Platters and sank in 11 metres of water. There were 73 people on board who were rescued by no less than four Lifeboats, those of Cemlyn, Cemaes and two from Holyhead.

Captain Waterston, a cautious man, was in charge of the Harrison steamer EDITOR, laden with cotton and sugar from Brazil in 1897. Thick weather for two days made him ensure that constant soundings were taken. Despite his extreme care his steamer ran into the rocks at Penrhyn Mawr where it quickly broke up. The crew of 27 abandoned into four ship lifeboats, which were helped ashore by the Holyhead Lifeboat.

The steamer BENHOLM, 1,438 tons, was sunk off Point Lynas in 1898 after being in collision with the streamer KLONDYKE, 10 of her crew drowned.

The Elder Dempster mail steamer DAHOMEY ran aground near North Stack in a fog in 1898. All passengers and crew were saved, 5 were landed by breeches buoy. Sixty tons of explosive cargo was brought ashore by tugs and the Holyhead Lifeboat transported the mails to safety.

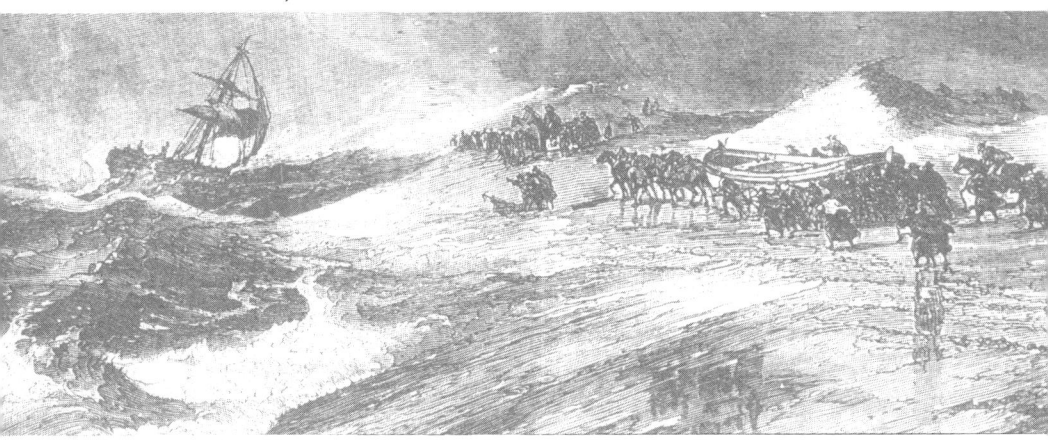

Failing to row the Lifeboat around Llanddwyn Island the Lifeboatmen collected a team of horses from Newborough to drag the boat through the dunes in 1852, to carry out a rescue from the beach at Malltraeth. The wooden ribs of the Greek brig ATHENA are still to be seen occasionally at low tide.

Shipwrecks since 1900

A terrific gale on 28th December 1900 drove ashore near South Stack one of the largest sailing vessels ever to be wrecked on any part of the Welsh coast. She was the iron clipper PRIMROSE HILL, a Liverpool 4 masted barque that was outward bound. Breaking loose from a towing tug off Bardsey the barque eventually came ashore and broke up within five minutes of hitting the rocks at Penrhyn Mawr. The waves were so ferocious that although the rocket brigade was quickly there they could do nothing to save the sailors washed into the sea. Only one man survived out of the 34 on board. The Court of Inquiry criticised the Captain of the tug for leaving the barque and made comment that the PRIMROSE HILL'S crew were inexperienced and insufficient for the voyage although there was no evidence to suggest that her loss was due to such inadequacy.

The crew of a Glasgow steamer STELLA MARIS had the dubious honour of being shipwrecked twice in twenty four hours and still remained alive to tell the tale. It happened in 1905 when their ship collided with the Spanish steamer ORIA off the Skerries. The STELLA MARIS sank, her crew jumped aboard the ORIA, which in a sinking condition, steamed for Holyhead. The ORIA sank half a mile off the breakwater, the crew of both ships abandoned into inadequate boats which managed to stay afloat long enough for all to be rescued.

Collisions at night or in fog have been the cause of many losses off the Holyhead coast. The steamer BLACKWATER, from Dublin to Liverpool, collided with the steamer WEXFORD in 1905, sinking the former. A steamer inward to Liverpool collided in thick fog with the outward bound CITY OF DUNDEE, holing and sinking the latter in 1908. A collision also caused the loss of the Dublin to Holyhead ferry ship SLIEVE BLOOM 4 miles off South Stack ten years later.

The Liverpool cargo steamer MAIORESE hit the North Stack in a fog in 1913. She was being towed back to Holyhead when she rapidly sank. The majority of the crew and all the passengers had been taken off by the Lifeboat, but whilst under tow the disabled steamer's bow suddenly plunged beneath the waves. The tug and Lifeboat then had a desperate task of searching for survivors that were swimming about in the darkness. 17 were picked up but 4 crewmen were lost.

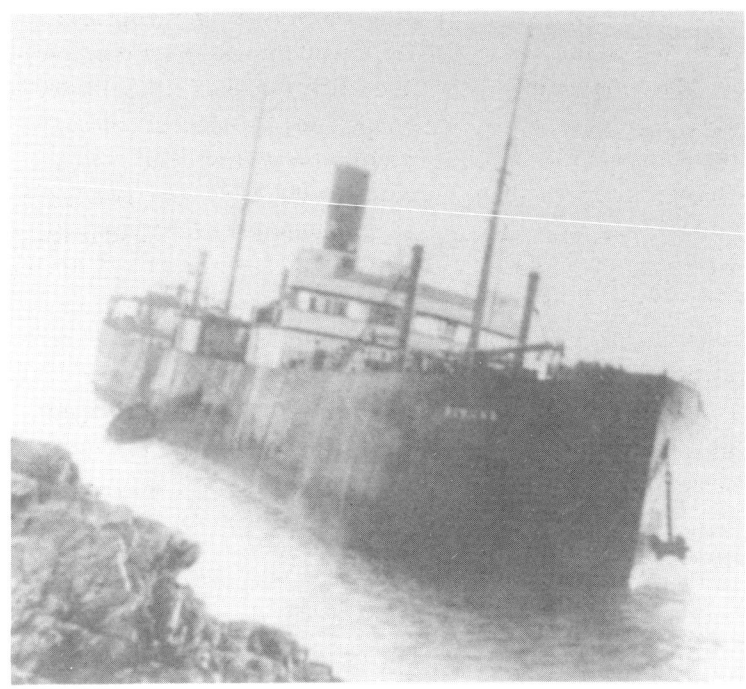

With a grain cargo intended for Manchester, the Norwegian steamer ASMUND hit the rocks near Porth Dafarch in December 1930. She was towed to Holyhead where she sank. The salvers had to race against time to pump her out before the grain swelled and split the hull. They failed, her hull now lies in Holyhead Bay. (Ian Jones Collection)

Enemy submarines caused many losses of both men and ships around the Anglesey coast during World War One. The Cardiff steamer CAMBANK was torpedoed 5 miles off Point Lynas in 1915. The merchant ship APAPA, 7832 tons, was sunk 3 miles off Point Lynas in 1917, and the following month the EARL OF ELGIN, 10 miles off the Caernarfon Bay lightship and the ADELA, 12 miles off the Skerries. In 1918 the TREVEAL was torpedoed off the Skerries, followed by PENVEARN 15 miles off Holyhead and FLORRIESTON 6 miles off South Stack, and the SEAGULL, 7 miles off Point Lynas. Other enemy victims the same year were the JANVOLD and DUNDALK.

A Lloyds report dated 3rd December 1930 stated: *"Norwegian ship ASMUND, Russia for Manchester, grain, ashore at Porth Dafarch, Holyhead. 3 landed by rocket apparatus, 16 by Lifeboat. Master, Officers and Engineers staying on board. Forepart lying on rock, for about 40 feet"*. The ASMUND (see photograph) was towed to Holyhead inner harbour where she sank. She was raised and towed into the bay where she sank for a third and final time.

Another Norwegian ship, HAVSO, was wrecked on the submerged rock Maen Piscar, off Trearddur, carrying scrap from Virginia to Birkenhead in 1937. Most of the 16 crew were in bed when the ship hit the rock and sank within 15 minutes. All were saved except for the ship's cat. The most terrifying experience befell the cook who clung to a floating hatch cover clung in the water for three quarters of an hour before his shouting alerted the Lifeboat that saved him.

There was an agonizing seven hour wait for rescue for the crew of the stricken coaster KYLE PRINCE. In big seas, the steamer's furnaces were extinguished. She drifted towards the Anglesey coast, her crew not knowing if an SOS had been heard. The Holyhead Lifeboat saved the crew and the derelict steamer broke up near Aberffraw.

Beacons and Lighthouse lights were deliberately extinguished to confuse the enemy in World War II.

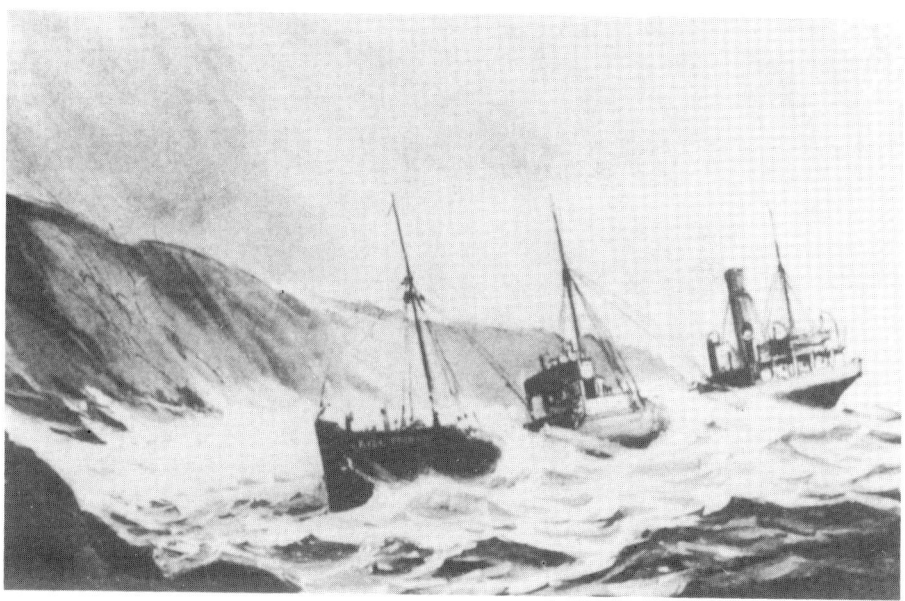

The Liverpool coaster KYLE PRINCE drifted helplessly towards the Anglesey coast in 1938. The crew were rescued by the Holyhead Lifeboat before the steamer hit the rocks near Aberffraw. (Brian Entwistle)

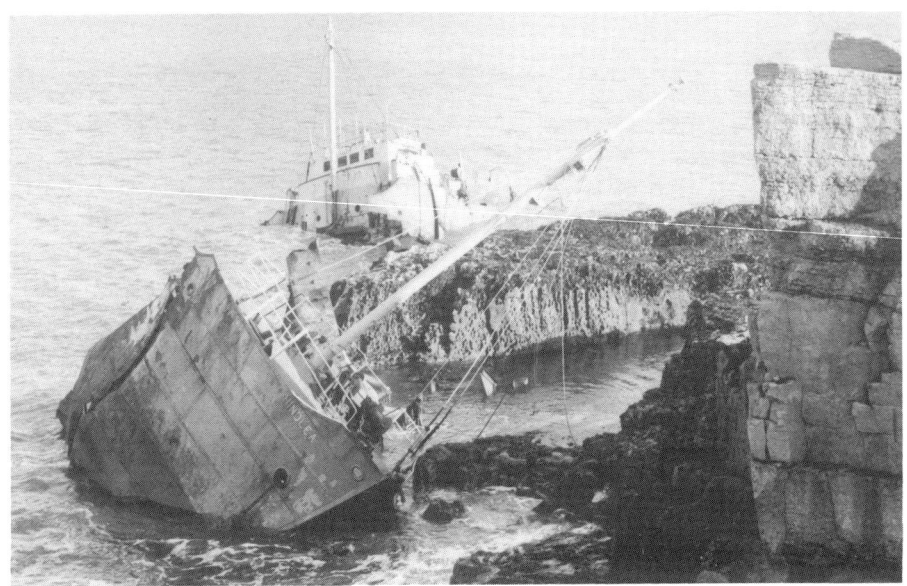

The Cardiff cargo ship HINDLEA II smashed into pieces on the rocks at Moelfre in an October gale in 1959, 8 men were taken off only minutes before, by Moelfre Lifeboatmen using a reserve Lifeboat. Coxswain Dick Evans was awarded an RNLI Gold Medal for this rescue. (Geoff Charles, National Lirbrary of Wales)

This was a hazard to allied shipping and caused the loss of the KYLE FIRTH which ran into the rocks at Penrhyn Mawr.

The summer of 1940 saw a variety of shipping losses in the Holyhead area due to enemy activity. The Admiralty patrol boat CAMPINA, a trawler of 290 tons, sank beyond the breakwater and a magnetic mine sank two more ships. The MEATH (or LADY MEATH) of the B & I Company carrying 781 cattle and 1008 sheep was blown up in the outer harbour as was the patrol boat MANX LAD that went to her aid.

Navigational difficulties caused two Canadian steamers to strand near Newborough in 1940. The EAGLESCLIFFE HALL was re-floated a few days after stranding but the WATKIN F NESBITT was cut up on the beach, the stern being refloated for reconstruction, leaving the forepart abandoned on the beach Ellerman line CASTILIAN, 3067 tons, ran aground and sank on the East Platters in 1943. Naval clearance divers have removed most of her live ammunition cargo.

The Cardiff vessel HINDLEA caused national headline news when she came ashore at Moelfre. It was just after midday on 27th October 1959, one hundred years after the ROYAL CHARTER disaster in almost the same spot. The HINDLEA radioed for assistance when she was drifting towards the rocks. She was only half a mile off and unable to make headway against the storm. Three quarters of an hour later the Moelfre Lifeboat was alongside and in huge seas took eight men off. Half an hour after abandoning to the Lifeboat the HINDLEA hit the rocks and immediately smashed to pieces. It was a brilliant rescue earning Coxswain Evans a gold medal, Mechanic Owen a silver medal and three bronze medals were awarded to the crew.

The heroism of the Moelfre lifeboatmen was displayed again in 1966 when the Greek vessel NAFSIPOROS got into trouble off the North Anglesey coast. A cyclone hit that part of the coast and the NAFSIPOROS was drifting, her propeller out of the water, in the 10 metre swell. Three Lifeboats were sent to her aid, the Holyhead Lifeboat and the Moelfre Lifeboat took off the majority of the crew. It was an extremely dangerous mission and nearly disastrous when a lifeboat from the stricken ship dropped out of its davits onto the Holyhead Lifeboat during the rescue. The NAFSIPOROS was later towed to Liverpool.

Since the 1970's the losses around Anglesey have been mainly commercial fishing vessels or private pleasure craft. In 1971 the motor vessel HOVERINGHAM II sank off Penmon Jetty, her upturned hull is to be seen at low water today.

The largest vessel to sink in recent times was the KIMYA (1800 tons) in 1991. Ferocious seas built up in two days of storm capsizing the tanker with its sunflower oil cargo. All 12 crewmen were on the bridge at the time and were thrown into the icy cold water. Miraculously 2 crew survived, being picked up an hour later by the RAF Brawdy Helicopter. The remainder of the crew were lost. The upturned hull of the KIMYA can still be seen today at low water off Aberffraw. The author cannot understand why regular merchant seamen do not keep dry suits to don in such circumstances. Such clothing, with the addition of a strobe light, would probably have saved their lives.

Lifeboats and Lifeboatmen

Prior to the formation of the RNLI monetary awards were given to persons who had successfully rescued life from shipwreck. The Druidical Society of Anglesey had paid out 161 in such awards during the years 1772 to 1821.

In 1809 Lloyds gave Holyhead a grant to maintain a Lifeboat. Although a purpose built Lifeboat was stationed there then, no records exist of its dimensions or what rescues it performed. Inspired into action after watching helplessly as 145 people drowned on the West Mouse rock in 1823, Frances Williams and her husband devoted the rest of their lives making sure such an incident did not happen again. The couple were the driving force in the formation of the Anglesey Lifeboat Association which achieved great success in establishing six Lifeboat stations. The Reverend James Williams was Secretary of the Association and was justly awarded an RNLI gold medal for a rescue in 1835. His son, Owen, was later a Coxswain of the Cemlyn Lifeboat, and he gained an RNLI award for towing a disabled schooner to shelter in 1853.

The Association's first Lifeboat station was at at Cemlyn in November 1828. It was a five oared Lifeboat nearly

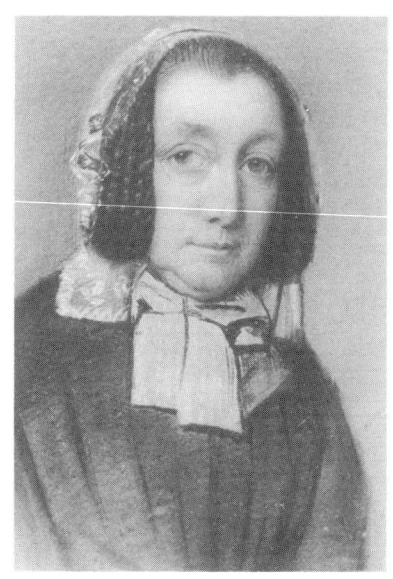

Frances Williams, founder of the Anglesey Association for the Preservation of Life from Shipwreck that established six Lifeboat stations around the Anglesey coast. (National Library of Wales)

8 metres long and 2 metres beam. The first Anglesey Coxswain to be awarded an RNLI gold medal was Captain William Owen for saving 11 men from the American ship PLUTARCH in 1835 using the Holyhead Lifeboat. This Lifeboat saved 124 lives between 1828 and 1857 when it was replaced with a new Lifeboat. The Holyhead Lifeboats have rescued 1,321 lives during 150 years of operation and at least 15 Lifeboats have been stationed there. It was Chief Coastguard Williams who persuaded the RNLI that one Lifeboat at Holyhead was not

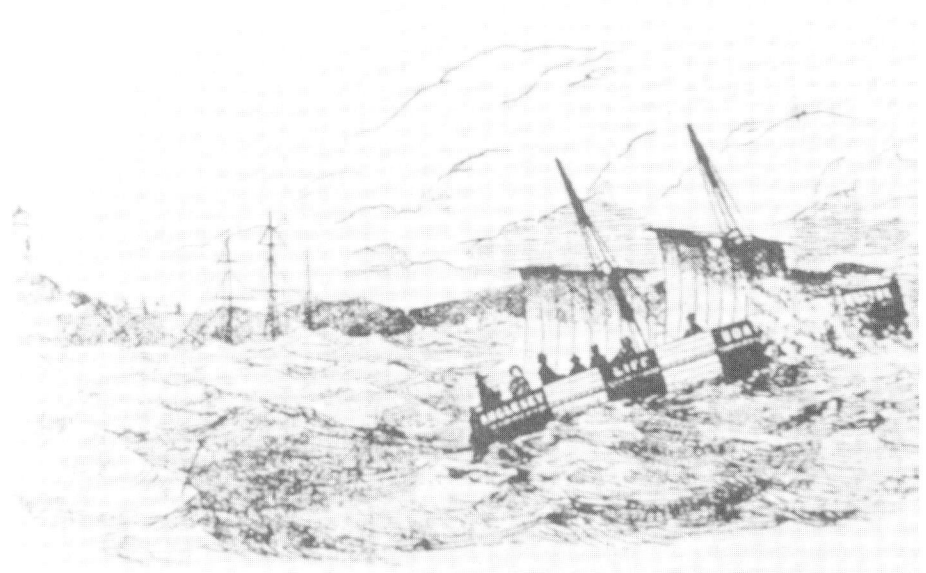
Contemporary drawing of an Anglesey Association Lifeboat drawn by Frances Williams.

sufficient for the work load and in 1890 a second station was established. Two years later there were actually three Lifeboats at the port. The third being the first operational steam Lifeboat DUKE OF NORTHUMBERLAND, capable of 9 knots, 248 lives were saved by this Lifeboat whilst she was based at Holyhead. One rescue in 1908 earned Coxswain Owen a gold medal. In 1966 further medals were awarded to the crew and a gold medal to Commander Harvey for their part in the NAFSIPOROS rescue.

Due to the difficulty of rowing the heavy Holyhead Lifeboat around the Stacks into the prevailing weather, it was decided to station a Lifeboat at Porth Rhuffydd. It was not a success and was there from 1891 to 1904 with only two service launches to its credit. The Association formed a Rhoscolyn Lifeboat in 1830 with a new Lifeboathouse built in 1878. The saddest of events happened in 1920 when 5 Rhoscolyn lifeboatmen were drowned whilst performing a rescue on the steamer TIMBO. They rest together in a grave at Rhoscolyn churchyard.

Rhosneigr had a Lifeboat station from 1872 to 1924, there were four Lifeboats during this time and uniquely all bearing the same name of THOMAS LINGHAM, 70 lives being rescued. Trearddur Bay now has an Inshore Lifeboat.

On the south side of Llanddwyn Island is Porth y Cychod also known as Pilots'Cove. It was here that the pilots to Caernarfon were based and they formed the heart of the Lifeboats that were stationed there from 1826. The Caernarfon Harbour Trust administered the Association Lifeboats from 1826 to 1840, this was replaced by an RNLI Lifeboat in 1861.

The RNLI opened Lifeboat stations at Bull Bay in 1868, Cemaes in 1872 and Beaumaris in 1891. The Penmon Lifeboat station was established in 1832 with an Association Lifeboat supplied by local subscription. Four subsequent Lifeboats were stationed here saving at least 116 lives until the motorised Beaumaris Lifeboat took over the area. The Beaumaris Lifeboat was established in 1891 but closed in 1895 to be re-opened in 1914 saving 127 lives up to 1968. It now houses an Inshore Lifeboat.

The actions of the Coxswains and Lifeboatmen at Moelfre have brought this Lifeboat station into prominence. Originally established by the Anglesey Association, Moelfre had its first joint RNLI Lifeboat in 1854. Since then more than 10 Lifeboats have been stationed there rescuing 646 lives between 1854 and 1968. In 1954 Coxswain John Mathews retired after 36 years service gaining 3 RNLI medals, 3 silver and a bronze. Since then Coxswain Richard Evans, is the only man in living memory to be awarded 2 gold medals, one for his part in the HINDLEA rescue in 1959, and the other seven years later for his part in the NAFSIPOROS rescue.

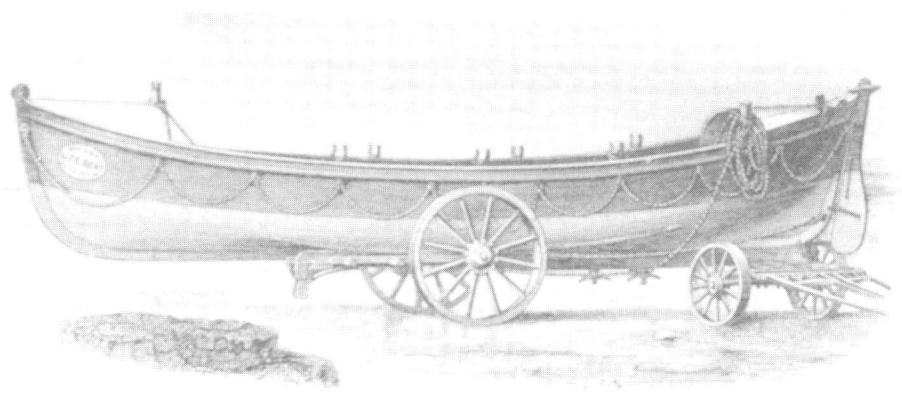

A typical rowing Lifeboat. This is a six oared Peake Lifeboat, the type that was stationed at Rhoscolyn from 1859 to 1872. (Tom Bennett Collection)

WRECK LIST

This is a chronological list of shipwrecks around the coast of Anglesey, and is confined to losses mentioned in the text. Losses in the Menai Straits will be included in another book. The numbers refer to the Wreck Chart to be found on the inside of the cover.

Abbreviations used for ship types;
BG = Brig, BGN = Brigantine, BQ = Barque, BQS = Steamer barque rigged, CUT = Sailing cutter, FER = Ferry, FRS = Full rigged sailing ship, K = Ketch, MFV = Motor fishing vessel, PS = Paddle steamer, RY = Royal yacht, S = Sailing vessel, SC = Schooner, SL = Sloop, SM = Smack, SS = Steamship,

Ship Name	Date Lost	Type	Location	Wreck No
BEAUMARIS FERRY	1325	FER	MENAI STRAITS N.END	
ABERMENAI FERRY	1664	FER	MENAI STRAITS	
MARY	1675 03 25	RY	SKERRIES	1
ANN	1710 09	S	IRISH SEA	
MOEL Y DON FERRY	1710 10 06	FER	LLANIDAN MENAI STAITS	2
TALYFOEL FERRY	1723 04 13	FER	CAERNARFON	3
BANGOR FERRY	1726	FER	MENAI STRAITS	4
LOVEDAY & BETTY	1740 12 31	BGN	RHOSNEIGR	5
PEARL	1760 11 03	S	CAERNARFON BAR SOUTH	6
CHARMING JENNY	1773	SL	CRIGYLL ROCKS	7
SILCOT	1778	S	CRIGYLL ROCKS	8
FAME	1785 09	BG	RED WHARF BAY	9
CORNELIA	1809	BG	HOLYHEAD	10
BRANSTE	1819 01 11	S	SKERRIES	11
FRIENDSCHAFT	1819 01 11	S	MALLTREATH SANDS	12
JANE	1819 01 18	BG	CAERNARFON BAY	13
WILLING MAID	1819 11 31	S	POINT LYNAS OFF	14
ROBERT BRUCE	1820	PS	CEMAES	15
TALYFOEL FERRY	1820 12 05	FER	CAERNARFON	16
ALERT	1823 03 26	S	WEST MOUSE	17
UNIDENTIFIED	1827 01 09	BG	SOUTH STACK OFF	18
HARLEQUIN	1829 04 28	S	HOLYHEAD	19
FAME	1829 04 28	S	HOLYHEAD	20
ACTIVE	1829 09 05	SL	HOLYHEAD	21
ROTHSAY CASTLE	1831 08 17	PS	DUTCHMANS BANK	22
IPHIGENIA	1832	S	HOLYHEAD OFF	23
MARTHA	1833 02 20	S	HOLYHEAD OFF	24
GEORGE	1833 02 20	S	HOLYHEAD	25
ACTIVE	1835 03 07	SM	CEMAES BAY	26
SARAH	1835 03 20	BQ	TWRYN DU POINT	27
PLUTARCH	1835 09 10	FRS	HOLYHEAD WEST	28
PANTHEA	1839	S	HOLYHEAD	29
GOVERNOR FENNER	1841 02 19	BQ	HOLYHEAD	30
NOTTINGHAM	1841 02 20	SS	ANGLESEY OFF	31
MONK	1843 01 07	PS	LLANDDWYN NORTH BANK	32
ALHAMBRA	1845 12 31	BQ	RHOSCOLYN	33
BROTHERS	1850 03 31	SM	PENMON	34
TOWN OF WEXFORD	1852 01 04	SS	HOLYHEAD WEST OF	35

Ship Name	Date Lost	Type	Location	Wreck No
ATHENA	1852 12 20	BG	LLANDDWYN, 1m NORTH	36
DIE KRONE	1852 12 26	BG	CAERNARFON BAR	37
JUNO 1	852 12 27	BQ	LLANDDWYN N BANK OFF	38
JOHN O'GAUNT	1854 01 16	FRS	TREARDDUR BAY	39
OLINDA	1854 01 26	SS	HARRY FURLONGS REEF	40
BONAVENTURE	1854 02 11	FRS	RHOSNEIGR	41
MINERVA	1854 08 29	SS	VICTORIA ROCK	42
SOUTHERN CROSS	1855 03 15	FRS	RHOSCOLYN HEAD OFF	43
ROYAL CHARTER	1859 10 26	SS	MOELFRE, LLIGWY	44
LIVERPOOL	1863 01	SS	POINT LYNAS.3/4mNNW.	45
LA PLATA	1863 01	BQ	POINT LYNAS, OFF	46
PAMELIA FLOOD	1863 01 20	FRS	ABERFFRAW	47
BRITANNIA	1864 03 11	S	RED WHARF BAY	48
EARL OF CHESTER	1867 10 27	FRS	RHOSNEIGR	49
EUPHRATES	1867 12	FRS	ABERFFRAW	50
LYDIA WILLIAMS	1867 12 01	FRS	SALT ISLAND,HOLYHEAD	51
BAYADERE	1867 12 01	BQ	HOLYHEAD LIGHTHOUSE	52
ATLANTIC	1868 01	BQ	ABERFFRAW	53
CYGNET	1870 05 12	SL	POINT LYNAS	54
ABBOTSFORD	1875 07 19	SS	WYLFA HEAD	55
MERLIN	1875 10 17	SC	HOLYHEAD BREAKWATER	56
NIAGARA	1875 06	FRS	PENRHOS FEILW	57
DAKOTA	1877 05 09	SS	EAST MOUSE ROCK	58
MONTANA	1880 03 14	SS	CHURCH BAY, HOLYHEAD	59
GILBERT THOMPSON	I881 03 05	BQ	WEST MOUSE ROCK	60
NORMAN COURT	1883 03 29	BQ	CYMYRAN, RHOSNEIGR	61
HOLYHEAD	1883 10 31	SS	IRISH SEA	62
ALHAMBRA	1883 10 31	BQ	HOLYHEAD 15m OFF	63
ADMIRAL MOORSOM	1885 01 15	PS	HOLYHEAD OFF.	64
JAMES KENWAY	1886 01 09	BQ	CARMEL PT.3/4m SOUTH	65
MISSOURI	1886 03 01	BQS	PORTH Y POST	66
LORD ATHLUMNEY	1887 06 04	SS	COAL ROCK, SKERRIES	67
GLEN GRANT	1889 02 11	BQ	PENRHOS HOLYHEAD	68
HERMINE	1890 06 16	BQ	PORTHYGARAN	69
GULF OF ST VINCENT	1890 07 19	SS	WEST MOUSE, SKERRIES	70
HUDIKSVALL	1890 11 20	BQ	CARMEL HEAD	71
MEATH	1892 02 01	SS	PENRHYN MAWR	72
MERSEY	1894 06 22	SS	PORTH RUFFYDD BAY	73
VALHALLA	1894 12 22	BGN	HOLYHEAD	74
TITANIA	1894 12 22	BQ	HOLYHEAD	75
JOHN WIGNALL	1894 12 22	SC	RED WHARF BAY	76
KIRKMICHAEL	1894 12 22	BQ	HOLYHEAD BREAKWATER	77
ANGLOMAN	1897 02 09	SS	SKERRIES, W.PLATTERS	78

Ship Name	Date Lost	Type	Location	Wreck No
EDITOR	1897 03 22	SS	PENRHOS POINT	79
BENHOLM	1898 05 19	SS	POINT LYNAS OFF	80
DAHOMY	1898 10 09	SS	HOLYHEAD,NORTH STACK	81
PRIMROSE HILL	1900 12 28	BQ	PENRHOS POINT	82
STELLA MARIS	1905 01 07	SS	SKERRIES 2m WEST	83
ORIA	1905 01 08	SS	HOLYHEAD BREAKWATER	84
BLACKWATER	1905 07 10	SS	SKERRIES 2m WEST	85
CITY OF DUNDEE	1908 10 04	SS	IRISH SEA	86
CAMBANK	1915 02 20	SS	POINT LYNAS 5mENE	87
APAPA	1917 11 28	SS	POINT LYNAS OFF NNW	88
EARL OF ELGIN	1917 12 07	SS	CAERNARFON LT 10m W	89
ADELA	1917 12 27	SS	SKERRIES 12m NW OFF	90
TREVEAL	1918 02 04	SS	SKERRIES	91
DJERV	1918 02 20	SS	SKERRIES OFF	92
PENVEARN	1918 03 01	SS	HOLYHEAD 15m NW	93
SEAGULL	1918 03 17	SS	POINT LYNAS 7m NE	94
SLIEVE BLOOM	1918 03 30	SS	SOUTH STACK 4m WNW	95
FLORRIESTON	1918 04 20	SS	SOUTH STACK 6m OFF	96
JANVOLD	1918 05 26	SS	IRISH SEA,28kmNW BAR	97
PALMELLA	1918 08 22	SS	HOLYHEAD OFF 22m NW	98
DUNDALK	1918 10 14	SS	SKERRIES 5m NNW	99
TIMBO	1920 12 03	SS	DINAS DINLLE	100
ASMUND	1930 12 02	SS	HOLYHEAD	101
HAVSO	1937 07 21	SS	TREARDDUR BAY	102
KYLE PRINCE	1938 10 08	SS	ABERFFRAW	103
KYLE FIRTH	1940 05 13	SS	PENRHOS POINT	104
CAMPINA	1940 07 22	MFV	HOLYHEAD	105
EAGLESCLIFFE HALL	1940 11 12	SS	LLANDDWYN, NORTH	106
APAPA	1940 11 15	SS	POINT LYNAS OFF NNW	107
WATKIN F NESBITT	1940 12 06	SS	LLANDDWYN NORTH OF	108
CASTILIAN	1943 02 12	SS	SKERRIES E.PLATTERS	109
HINDLEA	1959 10 27	MV	MOELFRE	110
NAFSIPOROS	1966 12 02	MV	NORTH ANGLESEY	111
HOVERINGHAM II	1971 01 28	MV	PENMON JETTY OFF	112
MAARTEN CORNELIUS	1971 03 19	MFV	SOUTH STACK HOLYHEAD	113
SALAZAR	1971 06 03	SL	RED WHARF BAY	114
JOSEPH W	1971 09 20	MV	POINT LYNAS	115
KIMYA	1991 01 06	MV	ABERFFRAW	116
KATY	1994 01 16	MFV	RED WHARF BAY 1m OFF	117

Book List

ANGLESEY & LLEYN SHIPWRECKS, Ian Skidmore, C.Davies 1979
MARITIME WALES VOL 1–16, Gwynedd Archives Service, Caernarfon
PLANS IN ST GEORGE'S CHANNEL–1748, Lewis Morris, Beaumaris 1987
SAILING DIRECTIONS OF THE BRISTOL CHANNEL, Wilson, London 1862
SHIPS & SEAMEN OF ANGLESEY, Aled Eames, Anglesey Antiquarian Society
SHIPWRECKS AROUND WALES VOL 1 & 2, Tom Bennett, Happy Fish 1992
SHIPWRECKS OF NORTH WALES, Ivor Wynne Jones, David & Charles 1973
THE GOLDEN WRECK, Alexander McKee, London 1970
THE MEMORIES OF SIR LLEWELYN TURNER, J E Vincent (ed), 1903
THE STORY OF A PORT, HOLYHEAD, D L Hughes and D M Williams, 1967
THE STORY OF THE HOLYHEAD LIFEBOATS 1828–1978, Jeff Morris, 1979
THE WRECK OF THE ROTHSAY CASTLE, Joseph Adshead, London 1834
WRECK & RESCUE ON THE COAST OF WALES, Vol 1 & 2, Henry Parry, Bradford Barton, 1969

Caernarfon and Denbigh Herald
Illustrated London News
Liverpool Daily Post
North Wales Chronicle
Port of Liverpool News
Sea Breezes
Transactions of Anglesey Antiquarian Society

For those interested in knowing more about Anglesey's maritime history, the places to visit are Gwynedd Archives Service at Caernarfon, Oriel Ynys Mon at Llangefni, Seawatch Centre at Moelfre and Anglesey Coastal Heritage Centre at Aberffraw. Early newspapers can be viewed at the National Library of Wales, Aberystwyth or at the British Library Newspaper Library at Colindale.

By the same author

FISHGUARD LIFEBOATS (Fishguard & Goodwick Ladies Lifeboat Guild) 1984
SHIPWRECKS AROUND WALES Volume 1, Happy Fish 1987 & Reprint 1992
SHIPWRECKS AROUND WALES Volume 2, Happy Fish 1992
WELSH SHIPWRECKS Volumes 1,2 and 3, 1981 to 1983 (Out of print)

Acknowledgements

I am grateful to the staff of Gwynedd Archives Service, the National Library of Wales and Ian Jones of Beaumaris for their help in collecting photographs and a special thanks to the printer and those involved in correcting, typing and typesetting the text.